C000196468

WISE EATING IN WARTIME

IMPERIAL WAR MUSEUM

First published by the Ministry of Information in 1943

First published in this format in 2007 by
Imperial War Museum
Lambeth Road, London SE1 6HZ
www.iwm.org.uk

Please note the information in this book was issued by the
Ministry of Information in 1943 and must not be taken as
Government or Imperial War Museum advice

Text as reproduced in this volume © Crown Copyright
All rights reserved. No part of this publication may be reproduced,
stored in a retrieval system or transmitted, in any form or by any means,
electronic, mechanical, photocopying, recording or otherwise without
the prior permission of the copyright holder and publisher.

ISBN 978-1-904897-70-5

Printed by Graphicom, Italy

Wise eating in wartime

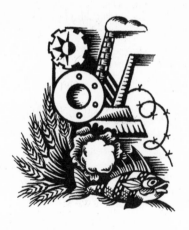

prepared for the Ministry of Food
by the Ministry of Information

WISE EATING IN WARTIME contains fifteen broadcast talks, on wartime diet for adults, given by Dr. Charles Hill. "The Radio Doctor," as he is known to millions of listeners, tells us how we can make the most of our rations, and keep our bodies tuned up to concert pitch by eating sensible, balanced meals. He takes us behind the scenes, showing the part played by various kinds of simple food in strengthening, warming, and refreshing the inner man. Everyone, from the housewife catering for a family, to the bachelor eating alone, will profit from Dr. Hill's cheerful and practical advice.

Contents

Acknowledgment is due to Hilaire Belloc and to Messrs. Duckworth and Co. Ltd. for permission to quote ten lines of Mr. Belloc's poem "On Food", from *Cautionary Tales*.

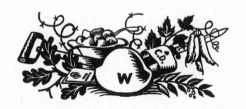

1. A little of what you fancy

To-day we are interested in food as never before. It's taken a war to make us interested, but that's by the way. In this little book I want to talk about some of the commoner dishes that turn up on our tables. But before I do that I want to remind you that you can eat the right foods in the right amounts of calories and proteins and what-not – you can run through the whole alphabet of vitamins – and still lack something important. That something of importance is *variety*.

Scientifically speaking, you could live only on milk and potatoes and cheese and something green and raw, and be healthy. As a matter of fact you would be bored to death and your digestion would suffer. Repetition day after day of the same foods, cooked and dished in the same way, is enough to drive a man to drink – and it sometimes does. I can speak feelingly on this. I liked Lancashire hot-pot, and I said so. But then it began to appear every Thursday as regular as clockwork. I don't like hot-pot nearly as much as I did. Bring a child up on rice pudding and in later life he'll loathe it. Familiarity has bred contempt, or something worse. Why is this?

First, a man's digestion is influenced by his state of mind. Monotony means poor digestion. Worry, too, may lead to indigestion, sometimes serious indigestion. Food for which you have an appetite is food that you digest better because of that appetite. And variety inspires appetite. A little of what you fancy does you good, because you fancy it, because you have an appetite for it; or because, having an appetite for it, you pour on it more digestive juice and digest it better. That's why foods which aren't essential foods – like sweets, or "afters", and cakes – have *some* place in our diet. They ring the changes. Another danger to digestion is worrying too much about what happens to the food inside you. I think it was Mark Twain who said that part of the secret of success in life is to eat what you like and let the food fight it out inside. That's half the truth.

Let your diet be scientifically sound and varied so that it tickles the appetite – and forget it when it's inside you. But remember that a diet which doesn't contain builders won't become a building meal simply because it's served by a pretty waitress. Food without vitamin C won't save you from scurvy simply because you're as hungry as a hunter.

The secret is to learn to fancy the right foods. But this is easier said than done. What stands in the way?

Well, first there's tradition, national tradition. It's not necessarily wrong, but when it's wrong it's difficult to move. Take for example the British habit of the Sunday joint. Hot on Sunday – cold on Monday – and if there's anything left, hashed or murdered on Tuesday. At least that was the pre-war routine in most of our households. Bang goes ingenuity and variety for the first three days of the week. Well, the war is damaging the Sunday joint tradition. And the Ministry of Food's education campaign is telling us of a thousand and one ways in which we can serve up the smaller bits, the odd bits of meat, attractively.

Secondly, there's use and habit. The wife has learnt to cook a few dishes and is content with them. She doesn't read the cookery book or the cookery articles. Someone has worked out that less than a quarter of this country's housewives use cookery books or read cookery articles. Mrs. Beeton's, rather like St. Paul's Cathedral, is known by everyone and visited by few. There's room for great improvement here.

I know that as a result of the war more and more people are eating out. But the vast majority of us still take most of our meals at home. We can't change our wives but they can change their ways, at least in giving their victims greater variety in their victuals. For variety means appetite – appetite means digestive juice –

digestive juice means digestion – and good digestion means good absorption, and that's what we want.

That Sunday joint

In the last chapter I was a little bit rude to the Sunday joint, blaming it for some of the monotony of English feeding – hot on Sunday, cold on Monday, and so on. I want now to probe a little more deeply the mysteries of that Sunday joint. We, in this country, aren't the biggest meat-eaters in the world. We come fourth, with New Zealand heading the list. Beef is our favourite. Before the war we ate more beef than pig meat, and more pig meat than mutton and lamb. But, of course, pig meat includes not only pork but bacon.

Here are a few figures. The poorest of us before the war spent about 1/1 per head per week on meat: $5\frac{1}{2}$ d. on beef, 4d. on pig meat and 3d. on mutton and lamb. The richest of us, those getting over £1,000 a year, spent 3/5 a head on meat. The great majority –

those of us who are neither rich nor poor but manage to rub along – spent 1/7 per head per week on meat. This gives us some idea of the reduction the war has meant – Not much is it? No, it isn't very much even if we bear in mind that the ration for children is half the 1/2 allowed for adults. These figures show that, as we pass up the income scale, so the amount spent on meat increases. It's not necessary, but meat, of course, is a tasty and appetising food. Over and above a certain amount, meat's a luxury.

Now for a word about its virtues. Here are a few points:–

(1) The edible part of meat is its muscle. Tender meat is mainly muscle with very little tissue in between – mainly muscle fibres. But the older the animal, the more it has worked, the more tissue in between – in other words, the tougher the meat. The woodcock is mainly a flier, the partridge is mainly a walker. Hence the doggerel – "If the partridge had but the wood-cock's thigh he'd be the best bird that e'er doth fly".
(2) The younger the meat the more water in the muscle fibres. "Calf meat is half meat," as someone once said.
(3) Freshly killed meat is tough, the *rigor mortis* – the death stiffness – is still there. Hang it, and the *rigor* passes off; and the meat becomes a little acid. This

acidity gives it a good flavour. That's why the flesh of hunted meat has a good flavour – from the acid due to the muscular exertion immediately before death. Soaking meat in vinegar for a short time improves its flavour by making it acid.

(4) The taste of meat is due, not to its protein – its building bricks – but to its extractives. The more mature the animal, the more its extractives and the better its flavour. But its food may influence its flavour. Wild duck is tastier than a farmyard duck. Mountain-fed mutton is better flavoured than turnip-fed mutton.

(5) What does cooking do? It loosens the fibres; it melts some fat and it evaporates some water. It makes the flesh more appetising. Lightly cooked meat is digestible; and overcooked meat isn't. Housewives please note.

Mutton is more easily digested than beef, and beef than pork. But under pork I don't include bacon. Bacon's very digestible, even by the youngest children. Breast of chicken is among the most digestible foods. Oh, shades of the past! Anyway, most of us can digest most meats most of the time. Lastly, the absorption of meat. Practically all its goodness is absorbed, and quickly. It's a well digested food.

Meat is supposed to arouse animal passions. This is

nonsense. Eskimos live mainly on seals and fish and game and eggs, and they're the most peaceful people in the world. Some vegetarians, on the other hand, are not so peaceful! What price Hitler? By the way, horse flesh is a good builder, though I've never tasted it. Our cat likes it anyway. But meat is a dear food, if a tasty one. As I have said before, meat's not essential. We need a certain minimum of builders, but they can be got just as well from milk or cheese or fish or eggs; good second-best builders are the pulses – beans and peas and lentils.

Offal good value for money

Yes, it's about offal and I promise not to make any more puns. I know it's often difficult to get, though it's been a bit more plentiful lately. But I'll tell you something of its virtues in case you can get a bit now and then.

Offal is about a third of the total weight of the animal. Under this heading we include kidneys, liver, sweetbreads, blood, heart, lungs, brains and tripe.

By the way, whenever I mention tripe on the radio I usually get at least one letter in which the word "tripe" is given quite a different meaning. But let that pass. Taking offal by and large, it's good value for money.

First, liver and kidneys. They are very solid organs stuffed full of food. For this reason they are sometimes difficult to digest unless they have been minced or, better still, well chewed. They are mainly building bricks of protein along with a little fat. There's only one snag. There's something in their protein which goes to make uric acid, the cause of grandfather's gout. So if you've a tendency to gout, lay off liver and kidneys. If you haven't, they're the goods.

The heart is a close-knit sort of organ: but if it is well chewed, most people can easily digest it. It's grand food – and what's nicer than a stuffed sheep's-heart? At first sight you might think that blood is a good food, even though you might not fancy it. As a matter of fact it isn't. It's four-fifths water – so blood's not much thicker than water after all. It's all right in black puddings, if you like black puddings, but it's nothing to write home about as a food. The same with lungs, or "lights" as the butchers call them. They're mainly wind, and goodness knows there's enough wind in our diet nowadays.

The term "sweetbread" covers two organs. It may be the thymus gland of the calf. That's a gland that's present in the human being in the early days but which shrivels up as we grow older. The other sweetbread is the pancreas. Now both of these kinds of sweetbread are among the most digestible animal foods we know. And they're good food except for the gouty. To him they are murder. At least to his big toe.

Now for the tripe, that tasty morsel of the North. No, the comedians are wrong. It's not liver struck by lightning or even boiled knitting. It's the stomach and intestine of the ox made clean and sweet by boiling. It's easily digested, though it hasn't much flavour. It's a bit pappy. But what's the tripe without the onions? Those who like it love it. Those who don't, won't touch it with a barge-pole.

Now for brains. They're rich in fat and in phosphorus, so necessary for bone. But oddly enough, they're not easily absorbed in the intestine, nearly half of them passing through and out at the other end. Apart from this, they are good food. But to eat brains isn't to grow brains or we could all belong to the Brains Trust, given the right diet.

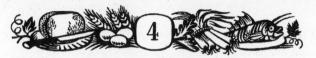

4

Fat fish and lean fish

Even in peace-time we weren't big fish-eaters in this country. For many people, fish hasn't enough flavour. They prefer their chops and steaks and roast beef – "they're tastier," they say. But tastiness, like ripeness, isn't all. Fish should be regarded as meat – as fish meat. It's a good building food. We can't get all the fish we want, for obvious reasons, but it's as well to know what's in 'em, if only to know what we're missing.

Let's classify our sea fish. Group one is fat fish – herring, salmon, eels, sardines, mackerel and sprats. Fat fish have abundant building bricks of protein and a good deal of fat. Weight for weight, fat fish like salmon – and that includes tinned salmon – are as nourishing as meat. And don't forget the slippery eel.

Fat fish contain some lime and some phosphates – the bricks and mortar of bone, and the stuff you need for healthy blood. They contain some iron, without which you can neither bloom nor blush. They contain some iodine – particularly necessary for children and adolescents for keeping their thyroid glands normal. They contain some vitamins, particularly vitamin A – the one which protects the body from eye and other troubles, and vitamin D – the one which protects from rickets and helps to build strong teeth. Even the humble bloater is rich in these good things. Fat fish is the best fish.

Now for the lean fish, for example cod, haddock and whiting. They contain roughly the same foods, except that they have very little fat, and less vitamins. They're said to be more digestible than fat fish, though cod's on the coarse side. Dried cod is simply cod with its water removed, and it is stiff with building bricks of protein. Smoked fish, such as smoked haddock, is dietetically as good as fresh fish and is just as well digested and absorbed as meat itself. If you cook your lean fish in fat, the finished article is almost as fatty as fat fish. For example, whiting fried in batter has almost as much fat as herring baked in vinegar.

By the way, don't come over all superior at the mention of fried fish and chips. It's not only very tasty and very sweet – it's first-class grub. That's true whether it's dished up with dignity to the Duke in his dining-room, or scoffed by the nipper from a newspaper spread out on his knees.

Let me say three things about fish I've said before: –

(1) It isn't a brain food – there's no such thing.
(2) Fish loses practically nothing in food value by

being canned or tinned or smoked. Let no one turn up his nose at tinned salmon.

(3) The herring is probably the best value for money of all building foods. Three herrings would give a man all the animal protein he needs for the day.

Now for fish offal. You know the value of cod and halibut-liver oil in giving vitamins A and D, the ones that all growing children must have. Fish roe, both hard and soft, is good food. It has a bit of everything – a lot of vitamins and a lot of phosphates. It's excellent for children. The millionaire's caviar is only the roe of sturgeon plus a lot of salt. Crab and lobster – they're fair food value, but they're not too well digested. Oysters – well, they make your mouth water; they may slip down like jelly – but their food value is poor. With oysters at 7/6 a dozen, it would cost you £2/5/- a day to get your protein from them. But, of course, they're not eaten for their food value. Mussels, winkles, scallops, are all juicy, but their food value is poor.

A word about coarse river fish. A fisherman friend of mine – and, when he's not telling me of the weight of the fish he's caught, I believe him – tells me that they are good eating. And you've only to look at him to realise that he knows what's good eating. Perch – they're good despite the thick skin. A lot of Lakeland perch are now being canned. Pike, when they are less than 5 pounds in weight, are very tasty, particularly baked and stuffed. Gudgeon and chub aren't very good eaters. By the way, to get the muddy taste out of these river fish, cook with mint or soak overnight in a solution of salt.

Lastly, tiddlers – but there I'm drawing a red herring across the trail. And, speaking of herrings, remember they give you the best return of all for your money.

The world's best food

Milk has a place of its own, as the world's second best food. Number one is breast milk. But we can't go on with that after the first year. Cow's milk is a nearly complete food with its builders of protein, its fat, its sugar, its lime, its phosphates, its good supply of several vitamins. True, it is poor in iron, it is poor in some vitamins, it lacks another. But apart from breast milk there's no other food to touch it.

Let's see how much we drank in this country before the war. On average, counting in everybody, young and old, we drank about $3\frac{1}{2}$ pints a week, or $\frac{1}{2}$

14

pint a day. Children had more, of course, and grown-ups less, but that was the average. Switzerland drank 9 pints per head per week; the United States of America 6. We can't be said to have been a milk-drinking nation, though as a result of a publicity campaign the amount consumed was rising. But it was still far short of the 6 pints per week per head of the population which the experts say we should on average consume.

Almost all of these $3\frac{1}{2}$ pints was being drunk at home, very little at restaurants and milk bars. Most of it was going into puddings. A lot was going in coffee in the case of richer people, and in cocoa in the case of poorer people. Then came custard and then breakfast cereals. But precious little was being drunk as liquid milk. What was wanted, then, was consumption of more and more milk as a drink. We have rather turned up our noses at milk. If we say that someone is a "milk-sop" we mean that he is weak and useless. If we talk of a "milk-and-water speech" we mean something pretty futile. The advertisements for beer may have led some people to think that it yields more strength than milk; that it's a man's drink; that milk is a little girl's drink. That's bunkum, of course. The strongest drink is milk. The war's an awkward time for increasing milk consumption, but a great deal is being done.

The Milk in Schools Scheme was here before the war. To-day getting on for 80 per cent. of our school children are drinking one-third of a pint of milk every day at school. But despite the fact that it's half price, or free if they can't afford it, there are still a few mothers who don't take advantage of the scheme. I know one who says that the child's tummy – it's an only child – is too delicate to digest milk. I don't believe it. Then there's a wartime scheme – an enormous social advance. The priority groups, the mothers and young children under five, are guaranteed their pint cheap, or if necessary for nothing. The other children get their half pint, plus their one-third of a pint at school. This scheme came in wartime and will, I am sure, stay in the peace which follows.

I have criticised many foods and so-called foods in my Kitchen Front talks, but never milk. Give twenty children an extra drink of milk a day and compare them with twenty without it. They are taller; they are heavier; they are healthier. Health can be bought in a bottle. An apple a day will keep no doctors away; but a pint of milk will, if it's given to children. Under 5's a pint at home, over 5's half a pint at home and a third of a pint at school. That's the stuff to give 'em. Take advantage of milk while it's plentiful.

Lastly, a word of warning. Germs like milk as well

as human beings. Milk should be pasteurised or boiled. In many areas it's all pasteurised. Where it isn't, scald it and keep it covered in a cool place. No boiling or pasteurisation affects the food value of milk to any extent. See your milk is safe and for health's sake drink it.

What can we do with milk?

The colder the climate, the more fat people eat – or want to eat. In Greenland, for example, they eat twice as much fat as we do here, and we eat three times as much as they eat in Japan. One reason is that, weight for weight, fat gives us over twice as much energy as starches and sugars. We can get twice as much heat from it. Fat gives us a nice comfortable feeling – we feel we've eaten something. But fat, and this is what limits our eating of it, is less digestible than other foods.

Butter and margarine are good and digestible fats. Butter is made from cream by churning it up so that the fat globules run together into a solid mass. Then the fat ripens, as they say, with the aid of a few germs, and becomes butter. It's four-fifths fat and one-fifth water. Butter's not easy to keep in hot weather, unless you do what they do in India, and melt it and boil it until all the water's boiled off, strain it through muslin and cork it up; then it will keep indefinitely. But butter's something more than just fat – just fuel. It's got two vitamins – A, which protects us from eye and other troubles, and D, which protects us from rickets and helps to build strong teeth. What's left of the milk when the fat is taken away is, of course, fat-free milk, or butter-milk. It's quite nourishing. Before the war it used to be thrown to the pigs, but it's much too good for them now.

Now for margarine. What a change there's been in it. Twenty-five years ago it was pretty loathsome stuff, with a tang you couldn't escape. To-day it's difficult to tell it from butter. It used to be made from the fat of the ox: to-day it's made mainly from whale oil and the oil of nuts and seeds, like coconut. It's a cosmopolitan mixture, for the whale oil comes from the Arctic and Antarctic, and the coconuts and seeds from the Tropics. Now, regarded as fuel, margarine to-day is as good as butter. But some of it lacks the vitamins – or did before the war. To-day the vitamins of butter are added to all margarine, with the result that it's just as good as butter, in fact it's got more vitamin D than butter. As for taste – well, I can't tell the difference.

What else can we do with milk? We can take it as liquid or powder. We can make cheese from it. We can make butter from it. We can drink it sour. A number of people write to me from time to time praising sour milk. One or two praise it as a cure for all the ills to which flesh is heir. Koumiss is a continental sour-milk preparation: it's made from mare's milk. Sour cow's-milk, made sour by adding a germ which acidifies it, or by adding the acid itself, is often drunk in this country. It's a regular article of diet in Russia. Some people prefer the taste. It's probably more digestible than ordinary milk in certain conditions of the tummy. And there's often a little alcohol in the milk, too, made by fermentation. Perhaps that's what gives it such a good name, specially amongst the teetotallers. But, to take it by and large, as Commander Campbell would say, it's just milk with a different taste.

Lastly, a word about dripping – Monday's breakfast for many of us. Its food value and its energy value are just as good as butter's. What it lacks are those precious vitamins. Nevertheless, it's good energy food, and not a scrap should be wasted.

7

Cheese – can you beat it?

Yes, cheese is our one and only topic in this chapter. Did somebody say that cheese isn't worth a full chapter? He's wrong. For all too long we've under-estimated the virtues of cheese in this country. We've too often treated this valuable food as a titbit – we've trifled with a serious subject.

But first of all, what is cheese and how is it made? When milk is clotted, the protein – that's the building bricks in it – becomes stringy and solid and the fat of the milk or most of it, gets caught up in the clot. The milk becomes curds and whey – the curds being the protein and the fat, and the whey mostly sugar and water. If it's cows' milk and the clotting is done by rennet, the curd is Cheddar cheese – after some water has been squeezed out. If cow's milk is clotted instead with an acid, like vinegar, less fat gets caught up in the clot and the result is a less fatty cheese. If goat's milk, partly skimmed, is used, the result is Parmesan cheese. If cow's milk is used, we get Roquefort cheese.

After the cheese has been squeezed, it's put in a cool place to ripen. If it's squeezed lightly, you get a soft cheese. If it's squeezed hard, you get a hard cheese. The ripening is done by germs – and the flavour depends on the germ which does the ripening. At present it's largely rule-of-thumb, and the germ depends on the district. Stilton is due to one germ and comes from one district. Gorgonzola is due to another germ and comes from another district. But the scientists are getting busy and putting in the germ they want – so they can make any kind of cheese anywhere. If the cheese is sterilised by melting and some salts added, we get a packet cheese which keeps very well.

Now taking cheese as a whole, a third is fat, a third is building protein, and a third is water. Two ounces of cheese contains most of the building bricks and fat of a pint of milk. That's the secret of the value of cheese. Beef is more than two-thirds water – cheese is only one-third. So, weight for weight, cheese contains twice as much nutriment as beef. A cheese of 20 lb. contains as much nutriment as a sheep's carcase of 60 lb.

Now the difference between different kinds of cheese is just a question of flavour – just a question of the different bugs or germs which do the work of ripening it. Parmesan is, or was, about twice the price of Canadian cheese, but its food value is no more than that of Canadian cheese – in fact it's slightly less. Of course, if cheese is taken just as a titbit at the end of a meal – well, flavour is everything – you've already had your food. But if cheese is taken, as it should be in these days of austerity, for the food value that is in it, then it should be remembered that the food value of the cheapest cheese is as good as that of the most expensive, and the food value of the imported is as good as that of the home-made.

What about its digestion? Now, I think that cheese has got a reputation for indigestibility it doesn't deserve. As I've said before, the cheese taken at the end of a big meal gives its flavour to the wind which may be belched up – and it takes the blame for what has gone before. It was the whipping-boy of the eats and drinks of the pre-war city banquet. It must be chewed, certainly – and a soft morsel is always more difficult to chew than a hard one. So a piece of hard, dry cheese is easier to chew than a soft piece. And it can often be grated. But taken by and large, and properly chewed, cheese is quite digestible. A piece of toasted cheese for breakfast and a cheese sandwich for tea – why not? There's nothing odd about it, really; it's just that we haven't the habit. After all, beer was the breakfast drink at public schools not so long ago. So why not cheese for breakfast? Cheese has much more to commend it.

Yes, I'm all for cheese. If I were allowed to say only three things about the Kitchen Front, I should urge something green and raw every day, I should praise milk and more milk, and I should preach the qualities of that food which contains much of what makes milk what it is – cheese.

Green leaves make rosy cheeks

Do you suffer from soreness of the gums, looseness of the teeth, anaemia, pains in the joints, bruises on the skin, gloom, irritability, fatigue and giddiness? If so, take our – no, not our pills. This isn't an advertisement for a patent medicine, after all.

Do you suffer from all these things? The answer's almost certainly "no," for these are symptoms of scurvy, that disease which used to worry sailors, explorers, soldiers in besieged towns, and all who lived for any time without fresh fruit or vegetables. Scurvy was Captain Cook's greatest enemy.

Scurvy is due to too little vitamin C – much too little. It's rarely seen to-day, though it was seen in a big northern industrial town in the last war. It sometimes happens in solitary bachelors and spinsters, living on their own, feeding themselves and doing for themselves. It has been seen in young men eating their mid-day meal in a city restaurant, and returning home to some warmed-up remains of a meal cooked hours before. Over-cooked or re-cooked food is the friend of scurvy.

But scurvy is so rare that the fear of it hardly troubles us. Scurvy's the whole hog, as it were. But the half hog isn't so uncommon. There are many who don't take enough vitamin C. They tend to be pale, to bruise quite easily, and to have poor complexions. An ounce of vitamin C is worth an inch of lipstick. It not only gives the skin a glow, but it helps it to heal. It keeps away infection, particularly from the so-called mucous membranes, such as the lining of the mouth.

"Well," you say, "where do I get my vitamin C?" Before the war you used to get it from your oranges, your lemons, and your grapefruit. You may have thought you got it from apples, but you didn't get much. Dietetically, apples are mostly skin and water (the Bramley Seedling, by the way, does contain some vitamin C). We got it from blackcurrants, rosehips, strawberries, raspberries, gooseberries and tomatoes, too – particularly from blackcurrants and hips. These are the fruits which were available then. Some of them you can get now, others are difficult to get. Eat all the fruit you can, but on the whole you'll have to go over to vegetables.

For a daily supply of vitamin C we must look first to raw vegetables – to raw cabbage-leaves, raw broccoli and raw brussels-sprouts, made up in salads. They are the cheapest and easiest way of making sure of regular daily vitamin C. Watercress and mustard-and-cress are good. Radishes and spring onions are not so good. Cucumber and lettuce are practically useless for vitamin C.

Most cooked vegetables contain vitamin C. They include broccoli, cabbage, cauliflower, kale, spinach, beetroot, runner beans and sprouts, but they must not be cooked too long or too much. The same with potatoes, turnips and swedes. For safety's sake, the green vegetables should be steamed for about 10 to 12 minutes. Put a little water in the bottom of the saucepan and cook with the lid on. Try your potatoes cooked in their jackets. Eat more of them, for vitamins' sake!

Now of all time, this is a time for salad vegetables. And I don't mean that slightly second-hand collection of wilting lettuce, with a suspicion of tomato and a chunk of cold potato, that sometimes masquerades as a green salad. It's better than nothing but it's not good enough. A salad should be freshly made, and if possible picked just before preparing. Go all out for the cabbage leaves, the watercress and the mustard-and-cress – all of them raw. To ring the changes, go in for endive,

25

chicory and finely grated carrot, and raw beetroot, and young dandelion, or nasturtium leaves. If you want a hot meal – well, sprinkle some pepper on it.

Remember what happened to those London kids who were given an Oslo dinner instead of a good old English dinner. They had milk, wholemeal bread, butter or margarine, cheese and raw green and other vegetables. They literally bloomed. From green cabbage leaves to red rosy cheeks. From dandelion leaves to rosebud lips. From raw green to bright red – that's a miracle the human body can manage. If you give it a chance.

Do we eat too much sugar?

Little girls *may* be made of sugar and spice and all things nice, though as a father of three of them I hae me doots. Anyway, all of us have sugar in our bodies if not in our dispositions. Starches and sugars are the cheapest energy food we have. I've lumped them together – no joke intended, by the way – for however we take our starch, whether in bread or potatoes or rice;

however we take our sugar, whether as sugar in our tea or icing on our cake (ha! ha!) all our starches and sugars have been turned into glucose by the time they get in our blood stream – that's the body's currency, so to speak. On average we get half our energy from starches and sugars. The poorer we are, the higher the proportion, for the simple reason that starches and sugars are cheap, particularly sugars. In Japan they get as much as four-fifths of their energy from starches and sugars.

For the moment I'll concentrate on sugars. Cane sugar is got from a special kind of grass, the sugar cane. Beet sugar comes from a root vegetable, the beet. These form the bulk of our ordinary white sugar. Maple sugar is tapped from the bark of a North American tree. Some people prefer the unrefined sugars, like Barbados or Demerara. But whether it's gran, or lump or castor – oh! blessed memory of the past – or brown or white, whether it's honey or barley sugar, or boiled sweets, it's sugar – fuel for the engine.

Treacle and golden syrup are by-products in the refining of sugar. They, again, are mainly sugars, with some iron and calcium as well. Toffee, by the way, is half sugar and half butter – or it should be. Many fruits contain their own sugar. Dates, figs, sultanas and currants, for instance – half to two-thirds of them is sugar. And prunes have quite a lot, too; they're nearly half sugar.

Now, do we eat too much sugar? Answer, "We do."
Sir John Hawkins brought the first load of sugar to
this country in 1563. Then it was a luxury. To-day it's
something of a menace. There is sound truth in the
quip, "Things sweet to taste prove in digestion sour".
A hundred years ago, everyone in this country consumed
about two ounces of sugar a week. Before the war, it
was over one pound a week per head, and still rising.

Why is it a menace? First of all, sugar has no value
other than the fact that it's sugar – that it provides
energy. Other energy foods, like bread, potatoes, have
got something else – some builder, some vitamins,
some salts. The danger of sugar is that, at least in ordinary
times, it tends to displace those other and better fuels.
It satisfies the appetite which should be reserved for
better things. Many doctors think that too much
sugar is responsible for some of our bodily troubles.

Well, the war has cut sugar down, and that's a good
thing, though it still leaves us a great deal. The snag is
that many of us have a sweet tooth and we like it. But
we can sweeten in other ways. To acid fruits, like
rhubarb, you can add sweet fruits, like dates. Now that
sweet biscuits are short, you can sweeten stale bread by
putting it in the oven for a few hours – when the
oven's on for another purpose. It should be warm but
not enough to brown it. Here you break down some

of the starch into a sugar. You can use saccharin: it's a harmless sweetener, though its energy value is nix. You can cut sugar out from your tea. Personally, I dropped it from tea some five years ago, and though I have a sweet tooth, I wouldn't give you a "thank you" for a cup of sweetened tea. But that's my funeral.

In moderation sugar's a good, cheap fuel. But there are better fuels and most of us eat too much of it.

Soup, soup, beautiful soup!

Someone once wrote to ask me why I never mention soup on the radio – good, hot, nutritious soup. She gives it, she tells me, to her boys every night when they come home from work. Isn't it good for them? she asks. The answer is, No! and Yes!

First – No! If it's a clear soup, made from meat cut up and simmered in water with the fat and the floating scum skimmed off, it's not much good as a food. The truth is that we just don't know how to get the goodness out of meat to make soup. We can boil out its flavour, its salts, its extractives as they're called, but we can't boil out those building bricks of protein that make meat the good food it is. To make it a meal, something must be added to the broth of meat or stock. You can add bones. By doing this you can boil out of the bones their gelatine. It's a building brick of sorts, but alone it's not much good. That goes for your calf's foot jelly as well. Secondly, you can add something to thicken the soup, like flour. Well, you've added starch and that at least gives it some energy value. But thirdly, and this is best of all, you can add vegetables. You can add lentils or peas, or potatoes, or turnips, or carrots, or cabbage, or cauliflower, celery or leeks. You can add cheese. You can add milk.

Now we're getting on to soups worth drinking because there's food in them. Boiling may kill a few of the vitamins in the veg., but it won't kill the salts. You'll notice that I mention lentils first. They make a grand soup and there's good grub in every mouthful. There's the No and Yes. No! to clear soups; and Yes! to soups with something added. Then why, you may ask, do people drink clear soup if there's no food value in it? The answer is, it's an appetiser. The flavouring and salts that have soaked out of the meat wake up your gastric juices and get them ready for what's to follow. As a Frenchman once put it, "clear soup is to a dinner what an overture is to an opera." I can't say

I like this comparison between drinking soup and the music of the band, but let that pass. Clear soup's no use to a hungry lad. His appetite doesn't need titillating. By the way, the meat you use in making soup may lose its flavour and become a bit leathery, but most of its goodness is still in it. So whatever you do, don't throw it away.

Is hot soup better food than cold soup? Well, I suppose it's better because we like it better. But the plain truth is, the food value is just the same. A food isn't necessarily an energy food because it's hot, else a glass of hot water would be a good meal. There's more warming food in a cabbage leaf with a dash of salad dressing on it than there is in a basin of clear soup that's scalding hot.

What about extracts of meat like beef extracts? They smell like meat. They've got its flavour. But they've very few of its building bricks, for we just don't know how to get them out of the flesh. Meat extracts are flavourers rather than foods.

The same applies to meat juices, whether you make them at home by squeezing meat in a lemon squeezer or by adding cold water and squeezing it through muslin, or whether you buy them in a bottle. They haven't got the full value of the beef or anything like it. They are often useful for invalids, though white of egg is a better source of builders and much cheaper.

Then there's beef tea. Its value, such as it is, depends on how you make it. What you mustn't do is to bring it to the boil quickly. It should be made in the cold and heated very slowly. It's useful for people on a liquid diet – no, I don't mean those who pour out their lunch in the local. But don't let's exaggerate its value even to invalids. It's an appetiser; and, to give you some idea of its food value, you would need nine pints of it a day to get your daily ration of protein. Just think of it, nine pints of beef tea!

But there is one way of getting the food value out of meat, though we don't use it in this country yet. It's by drying meat to a powder. Yes, I know it sounds like sacrilege to shrivel a juicy steak to a powder; but dried meat would take up less shipping space than meat in the raw, and we are going into the question of importing a high-grade dried meat from U.S.A., where it is being used already.

There then is the story of soup. Meat may flavour it, but it's the other things in it that make it worth drinking – the lentils, the peas, the turnips, the swedes, the celery or the leeks and – dare I make your mouths water? – onions when you can get them.

Soft drinks and hard drinks

Next I want to talk about drinks, soft and hard. First, everybody's drink – water. I know some people boast that they use it only for cleaning their teeth, but they take it all the same both in their drinks and in their eats. Two-thirds of the body weight is water, and growing young men or women need at least a couple of pints a day to replenish what they lose. If they are doing hard, physical work or taking a lot of exercise, they need much more. Their thirsts will tell them what they want.

There's no danger of drinking too much water. Most of us could do with just a little more water than our thirsts suggest. And don't forget the value of a glass of water, as soon as you get up in the morning, in helping the bowels to do their job. As for minerals, in which young people delight, their food value is nil or nearly nil. If they're fizzy, that's carbon dioxide gas under pressure. If they're sweet, syrup has been added, and so on. The food value – napoo.

Now for tea, mother's standby at all hours of the day and night. A century ago our tea came from China;

now it comes mostly from India. I haven't the cheek to tell you housewives how to make it, but please make it as soon as the water comes to the boil, and please don't let it stand for longer than five minutes.

What does it do for us? Well, it contains caffein, and caffein is a stimulant. It clears the head, it drives away that sense of weariness and it keeps us awake. One often heard bogey-men's stories of what tea can do to us, of what the tannin in tea will do to meat in turning it to leather, and so on. Don't you believe it. Most people of ordinary digestion can take properly-made tea two or three times a day – yes, even with a meat meal – without the slightest harm. I know some people say tea sends them all of a dither, but those people are usually all of a dither anyway.

As with tea, so with coffee, though it's said we don't know how to make it in this country. The food value of tea and coffee is precious little. They are stimulants, and in this weary world of ours we need stimulants. Cocoa, by the way, is hardly a stimulant at all. But it has some food value, though not a great deal. To give you some idea, you would need 75 cups of cocoa a day to give you the energy you need. Of course, cocoa made with milk is a different story: there, the goodness is due to the milk. So the moral is, don't think you are feeding your young people

34

when you give them tea or coffee made with water. But you will refresh them, particularly after a long day's work.

Now for a word about a drink which is not a stimulant, alcohol. Yes, I repeat, alcohol is not a stimulant. It's a depressant. It blunts the higher centres of the brain. True, it may damp down your worries; but it also blunts your self-criticism, it weakens your self-control, it impairs the accuracy of your skilled movements. True, it is a food that's quickly absorbed, but it's a very expensive way of taking your food – and we don't ordinarily need to absorb our food at top speed. And alcohol doesn't warm either you or your young people up on a winter's night. That's a snare and a delusion. It does make you feel warmer, by increasing the rate at which you lose your body heat. The fact is it makes you colder.

Let me sum up. Water we must have, and most of us might well drink more. Ginger-pop and the like have little or no food value. Tea and coffee have no food value, but they are grand refreshers and stimulants. Cocoa has some food value, and a lot when made with milk. Alcohol is not a stimulant but a depressant. But don't think that a liquid can't be a food, for food number one is a liquid – milk, the best food and drink bar none; particularly for those who are still a-growing.

Menu for the ideal meal

Many good foods are named after the places they come from, or are supposed to come from, just as many good schools are named after the roads in which they are situated. There's Brussels sprouts, and Jerusalem artichokes. There's Cheddar cheese, and Ostend rabbits, and Eccles cakes, and French pastries, to say nothing of Bath buns and German sausages.

Then, there's the Oslo breakfast. It isn't really a breakfast; it's a meal you can take for breakfast, dinner, or tea. And its only connection with Oslo is that it was first tried out in an Oslo school. It reminds one of the May week at Cambridge, so-called because it's held in June and lasts a fortnight. Now, the Oslo meal isn't a good meal just because it's foreign. I know that some musicians add Poposki to their names because they think we will like them better if we think they're foreign. There are restaurants which describe their dishes in French, perhaps so that we will fancy that they're better than they are. But the Oslo meal is good British food – none better.

Here it is. National or wholemeal bread, milk,

cheese, butter or margarine, and uncooked salad vegetables. How's that for a meal? It's cold, yes. But a meal isn't good because it's hot. And a hot meal doesn't give us heat to any amount which matters. There's no meat in it; but all the builders you can possibly need are in that cheese and milk and bread. Cheese, you'll remember, contains all the builders and most of the fat of milk. Milk is strong drink number one, and rich in builders and nearly everything else. And the National Loaf contains some builder as well as vitamin and iron. There's energy in the Oslo meal; and if there's not enough, you can fill up with potatoes to your heart's or your stomach's content. There's vitamins in it, particularly in the margarine, the bread, the milk and the uncooked salad. The Oslo meal is precious near the ideal meal.

You've heard what happened to the children who were put on the Oslo meal for dinner, and afterwards compared with the children on the good old English meat and two veg. with a pud. as padding. The Oslo kids felt fitter and they looked fitter – clear-skinned, bright-eyed, and full of vigour. They did better at play and at work. The Oslo meal's *better* than the hot dinner, and that goes for both children and grown-ups. Please, please don't think that veg. that are steaming are better than veg. that are stone cold. They're probably worse: if they're overcooked, they're certainly worse.

By the way, there are variations that you can make in this meal. Obviously the grown-ups can't have the same amount of milk as the children. They can make up with a bit more cheese. You can add potatoes and cut down the amount of bread. Don't forget the virtues of the humble spud – energy, builder, and vitamin food. You can ring the changes in the salad vegetables. There's the tomato with its vitamins A and C. The carrot – here it's mainly vitamin A. Then there's the old gang, watercress, mustard-and-cress, broccoli tops and cabbage leaves; and my old friend, the dandelion leaf.

But, if the children have the cheese, the milk and the salad veg., they're having the best food that this world can give, in peace-time as well as war-time. This is an old story, I know, but I must repeat it until it's not only believed but acted on. If you can't tear yourself away from the hot dinner, then have an Oslo tea. Cheese, remember, is good food, whether it's taken at dinner-time, at tea-time or even at breakfast-time. Have you ever tried a bit of toasted cheese at breakfast? It's lovely.

How to feed a fever

I must start this chapter on Food for the Unfit with a word of warning. Don't let us exaggerate what food can do to cure disease. It plays its part, certainly. But in most diseases it's a small part. It isn't a panacea for all the ills to which flesh is heir.

The human mind is apt to jump at the simple explanation, and at the simple cause. We hear it said, for example, that the inflammation has gone in instead of coming out, that an illness dates from falling down the stairs a month ago, or the shock of seeing a dog run over a week ago. We are apt to exaggerate as well as to over-simplify, due in part to our lack of knowledge of how the body works, though sometimes it's due to a glowing pride in our own ailments. You know how superior troubles of the heart are to disorders of the stomach, at least in daily conversation; how our pneumonias are nearly always double; how our friends have been told by their surgeons how rare, how interesting was the tangle they discovered in peeping inside them. And so it is with food. We are apt to blame it and to praise it too much for what it does when we are ill.

First, our food in fevers, and by fever I mean all cases of temperature of any duration, and not merely fevers that take us to the fever hospital. I mean your 'flu, and your colds, as well as your measles and your mumps. In feeding fevers there has been a revolution. For centuries, in fact, right back to the time of the Greeks, starvation was the treatment for fevers. The temperature was due, they thought, to an irritation of the gut. Therefore, they said, starve the patient and rest the gut. Actually they fed him on wine and barley gruel – not bad for starvation. Then, in the middle of last century, came the revolution. Starving fevers was replaced by feeding them, and that is what is done to-day. The fever patient is fed with fluids or semi-fluids to the limit of his digestive capacity. Mind you, a food's none the less a food because it's liquid. But every liquid isn't a food.

Here are the rules for feeding, when there's no doctor in attendance, as for example, if you have a cold. Plenty of starchy or sugary foods. I mean, for example, rice or semolina, and mashed potatoes with gravy. Drink milk, egg and milk, and milk flavoured with tea. Within reason eat what you fancy, if you have got it. For breakfast or tea, make it bread and milk or porridge and a scrambled egg. For dinner mashed potatoes and gravy and milk pud., and some steamed fish if you can get it. If the appetite's poor, titillate it with some beef tea, unless there's diarrhoea. Don't drink beef tea in diarrhoea.

If you are chesty, take your food hot. If there are colly-wobbles in your tummy, cut out the solids but take plenty of warm water. Keep off meat while your temperature is up. And drink plenty of water. Do fevers need alcohol? At one time a little brandy was the commonest medicine for the patient and some-times for the nurse. Those days are gone. A man used to alcohol may need it to get him to sleep. The others don't need it in fever.

By the way, let me add a special word on milk, that standby in both sickness and health. True, there is some milk available as an additional ration in cases of sickness, but it's very, very limited. Your doctor *can* prescribe extra milk for you if you are suffering from one of quite a short list of complaints. But, unless your illness is in this list, there is no milk for you; so don't go on worrying your doctor for a certificate. The poor doctors to-day are hard pressed. Spare them wherever you can, particularly by not asking for certificates which you don't need, or to which you are not entitled.

Food fairy-tales

Does eating crusts make your hair curl? Does drinking egg water give you warts? Does an apple a day keep the doctor away? It's questions like these that are always cropping up in my post. Let me deal with some of them. What truth is there in these simple and attractive wrinkles?

"An apple a day keeps the doctor away." Well, what's in an apple? It's over four-fifths water. And no doctor is frightened of water. The only food of any real value in the apple – if it's not a sour one – is a spot of sugar; a few grains in the ordinary apple, amounting to one-eighth of the apple by weight. For the rest there's a tit-bit of roughage, a spot of acid, a suspicion of fat and builder. Dietetically, the apple's a skinful of water with a trace of vitamin C. Only the Bramley Seedling contains much vitamin C. Apples are pleasant, they are refreshing, they help to clean your teeth. But they're as much use in keeping a doctor away as a roaring pneumonia. Now, if you say, "Something green and something raw every day keeps the doctor away," you're nearer the truth. That's if you *want* to keep the doctor away.

"You get warts if you drink water in which an egg has been boiled." Now, how can you? Warts are little overgrowths of skin. The egg-shell is mainly carbonate of lime. Lime does you no harm in small amounts. And it has nothing to do with the growth of your skin. This is an old wives' tale with a vengeance. And by the way, there's no real difference between eggs with dark shells and eggs with light shells. There's no justification for the belief that dark-shelled eggs are richer than light-shelled eggs.

"National bread has a germ in it. Can this germ cause disease?" That's a quotation from a letter to me. Confusion here arises because the word "germ" has two meanings. When you catch tonsillitis, it's germs – bacteria, bugs – which are wallowing in the cracks and crevices of your tonsils. When we speak of the germ of wheat we mean, not bacteria, not disease germs but the germinating part of the wheat grain, the part which grows to form the new plant. It's a bud not a bug.

"Raw vegetables give children worms." They don't. It's worms that give children worms – worms taken by the mouth with the food or water we take in. Certainly unwashed vegetables, like other unwashed foods, may carry worms. But the vegetables themselves don't give you worms. In short, wash your green vegetables and salads.

"Crusts make your hair curl." Well, well, well. Try it and see. Think of the poor perpetrators of permanent waves if this were true. But, alas, it 'aint.

"Oranges and other fruits give children acidosis." Well, I won't worry you with details of acidosis, which was all the rage years ago. But I can assure you that because fruit tastes tart, because it contains acid, it doesn't mean that it gives children acidosis. Don't deprive them of any blackcurrant juice you can get because of this bogey.

"I don't feel I can take live vitamins." someone wrote. We must get clear that vitamins aren't alive. They are chemical substances which are present in many natural foods, and without which the body can't be healthy. Many of them can now be prepared by the chemists in their laboratory. They aren't alive; and in any case, a digestion which can take Stilton cheese when it's all "alive" wouldn't be disturbed by a few vitamins – if they were alive.

Those are some of the myths which our gossipy friends, the astrologers of dietetics, would have us believe. We no longer fall for the one about the gooseberry bush and the part it plays in our birth rate. We no longer believe that for a child to pick dandelion leaves is to stimulate its kidneys beyond hope of control. So don't let's be taken in by the fairy tales of feeding.

A matter of taste

This chapter I want to start with a poem. It's by Hilaire Belloc: –

> "Alas! what various tastes in food,
> Divide the human brotherhood!
> Birds in their little nests agree
> With Chinamen, but not with me.
> Colonials like their oysters hot,
> Their omelettes heavy – I do not.
> The French are fond of slugs and frogs,
> The Siamese eat puppy-dogs.
>
> And all the world is torn and rent
> By varying views on nutriment."

Well, what are these varying views on nutriment? First, I think, comes vegetarianism: it's a *different* view, held by a good many people. Some of the arguments for it are moral and aesthetic: that animal food is revolting, that meat-eating involves cruelty in the killing of animals. That's a matter of conscience rather than of physiology. The second argument for it is that it works. Whether you look in the fields of physical or intellectual activity, you find vegetarians among the giants. There are three main varieties of this system. There are the fruitarians, who eat fruit only. There are the vegetalians, who eat fruit and vegetables only. And there is the normal vegetarian who eats, in addition to fruit and vegetables, milk and its products, butter and cheese and eggs.

Now, fruitarianism – there's no sound argument for this. The ape may live only on fruit, but it doesn't follow it's good for man. To obtain the energy you need and the builders you need from fruit, you would have to eat simply enormous quantities. And the builders in fruit, such as they are, are not really good enough for man – at least as his only builders. Neither your stomach nor your purse is big enough, even in the days of plenty.

The vegetalian lives only on fruit and vegetables. Here again the vegetables are too bulky, and the builders aren't good enough, though in beans and lentils they are pretty good. It's not a satisfactory diet.

Thirdly, the normal vegetarian. On dietetic grounds there's nothing at all to be said against excluding meat from the diet, provided you replace it by cheese and eggs and milk. I don't like the meatless diet every day because I find it insipid: it lacks flavour and taste. But the fact remains that you can get from cheese and milk and eggs all you can get from meat. You can be vegetarian and absolutely healthy. It's all a matter of taste.

Now for one or two fads. There's the unfired food fad. Its adherents argue that no animal cooks food. Man is an animal, therefore man should not cook. Well, the other animals don't talk or read or wear clothes. Is that any reason why man should copy them? The fact is that cooking improves the flavour and digestibility of the food. It often makes it safer. It gives it variety.

Then, there's the fad of incompatibility – that some foods should not be eaten with others. In Canada it is widely held that you should not drink milk at a meal at which you have stewed fruit. The acid of the fruit would curdle the milk. Well, the acid of the stomach is going to do it anyway. It's just a fad.

Then there's the system of dieting which says, "You mustn't eat building food, like meat and cheese, at the same meal as sugar and starch. Meat and potatoes is a dietetic crime. Those much-married foods, bread and cheese, must never be seen together!" Dietetically this is bunkum. It's the only word for it. The only thing to be said in its favour is that it may make some people eat less. The prosperous business man found himself cut down to a glass of milk and a little fruit or salad. He ate less and he had more vitamin foods. He was the better for the starvation: the incompatibility, so-called, had nothing to do with it.

Lastly, is there anything in the slogan, "Never drink at meals," or in the other one, "Never drink between meals?" Of course, it's wrong to wash food down with copious drinks at a meal-time. The saliva doesn't get a chance to do its work. But for the ordinary man drinking ordinary amounts of ordinary drinks, particularly water, the fact is that it doesn't much matter whether you drink with your meals or between your meals. Please yourself – there's some welcome advice for you.

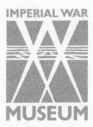

IMPERIAL WAR

MUSEUM